HOT STONE MASSAGE

The Essential Guide To Hot Stone And Aromatherapy Massage

Alison Trulock

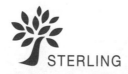

STERLING

New York / London
www.sterlingpublishing.com

Library of Congress Cataloging-in-Publication Data
Trulock, Alison.
  Hot stone massage : the essential guide to hot stone and aromatherapy massage / Alison Trulock.
    p. cm.
  Includes index.
  ISBN 978-1-4027-5564-4
1. Massage. 2. Hydrostone therapy. 3. Aromatherapy. I. Title.

RA780.5.T78 2008
615.8'22--dc22

                                    2007052564

10 9 8 7 6 5 4 3

Published by Sterling Publishing Co., Inc.
387 Park Avenue South, New York, NY 10016

© 2008 by Sterling Publishing Co., Inc.

Distributed in Canada by Sterling Publishing
c/o Canadian Manda Group, 165 Dufferin Street
Toronto, Ontario, Canada M6K 3H6
Distributed in the United Kingdom by GMC Distribution Services
Castle Place, 166 High Street, Lewes, East Sussex, England BN7 1XU
Distributed in Australia by Capricorn Link (Australia) Pty. Ltd.
P.O. Box 704, Windsor, NSW 2756, Australia

Photos © Shutterstock.com

Printed in China
All rights reserved

Sterling ISBN 978-1-4027-5564-4

For information about custom editions, special sales, premium and
corporate purchases, please contact Sterling Special Sales
Department at 800-805-5489 or specialsales@sterlingpublishing.com.

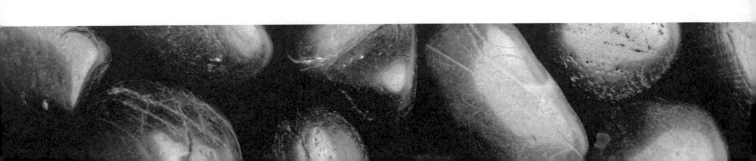

CONTENTS

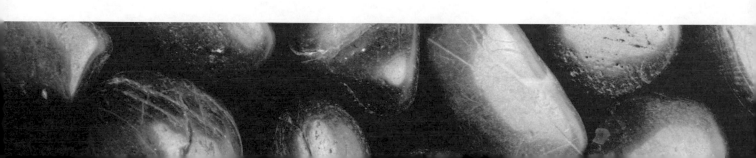

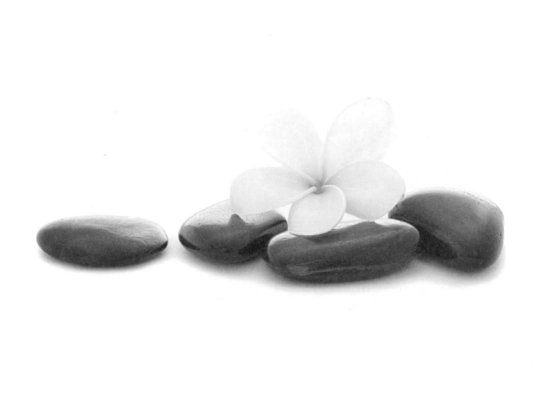

INTRODUCTION

TOUCH AND FEEL: MASSAGE AS A HEALING TOOL

There's a lot of pressure that comes along with everyday life. Pressure to perform at work, maintain healthy relationships, and spend enough quality time with your family and friends. All of your commitments leave you little time to relax and take a breather, which all adds up to a lot of tension that you carry around with you. This not only leaves you feeling tired and stressed, but has the potential to make you more prone to illness. With so much to do and see, who needs that kind of extra weight?

However, there is a particular kind of pressure that *is* good for you. To many people, massage may be something reserved for a special occasion or only when a little "pampering" is in order. But, as massage has entered the mainstream and more long-term studies have been performed on its benefits, more and more people are turning to massage to relieve mental and physical stress and to alleviate symptoms of some common conditions—not just as a way to feel good once in a while. Massage is the ideal way to effectively release the buildup of tension in your muscles, leaving you feeling refreshed, rejuvenated, and ready for anything.

Massage is the practice of applying pressure, tension, motion, or vibration to the soft tissues of the body (which includes muscles, tendons, joints, and ligaments) with the goal of relaxing these areas. Massage has been shown to have a positive effect related to the healing of injuries, the reduction of mental stress, the management of pain, and the improvement of circulation. Different types of massage have been developed to target particular areas or produce specific results, such as in sports; Swedish; shiatsu; deep tissue; and the focus of this book, hot stone massage.

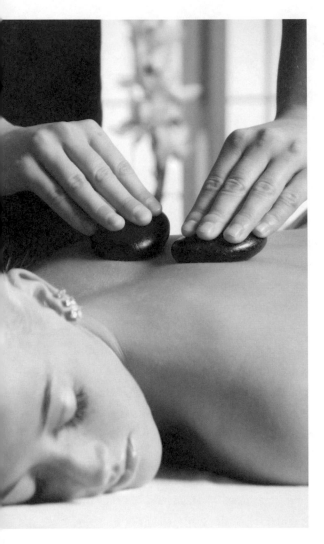

Keep in mind that every person has different needs and reacts differently to massage, even from one massage to the next. Make sure you're aware of any special conditions before you begin the massage, and be ready to adjust the massage as needed per your partner's specifications. Massage works wonders on most people, but note that if any of the following describes you, massage may not be recommended, and you should consult with your physician before undergoing massage therapy:

- If you have an infectious skin disease, rash, or open wound
- If you have just undergone surgery
- If you have just had chemotherapy or radiation
- If you are prone to blood clots or have heart disease
- If you are pregnant (Massage can be very beneficial during pregnancy, but it should be performed by a massage therapist trained in pregnancy massage.)
- If you have bruises, inflamed skin, unhealed wounds, tumors, abdominal hernia, or a recent fracture (These areas should not be massaged.)
- If you are taking medication that may cause skin to be hypersensitive
- If you are diabetic (Diabetics have decreased sensation in their extremities, and should be monitored closely during hot stone massage.)

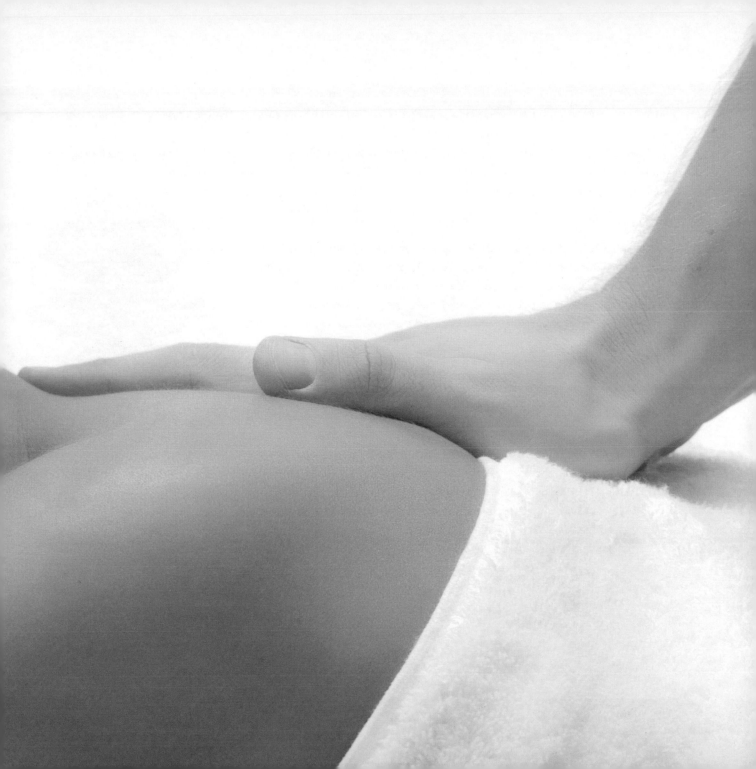

Feeling Good Is Good for You: The Benefits of Massage

Stress isn't just all in your mind. The effects of stress are felt throughout the body. It can manifest itself in the form of headaches and upset stomachs, as well as a general feeling of fatigue. The body and the mind are intricately linked, and because massage relaxes the body, it also relaxes the mind. Regular "doses" of massage will help you feel more peaceful and balanced and ready to handle stress.

In an age where writing a prescription is often seen as the cure for anything, massage provides a natural and effective alternative for treating some common maladies.

- Massage improves circulation. The increased blood flow improves the skin.
- Muscles that have been overworked are softened by massage.
- Cramping and spasming can be reduced by massage, and joint flexibility is increased.
- Massage releases endorphins (the body's natural painkiller)—which are also released during exercise, providing that energized feeling you get after a workout.
- Massage promotes healing in the body, which can reduce recovery time after an injury or after a workout.
- Overall, simple touch is one of the best, and probably most overlooked, healers. Think about some common behaviors when people are feeling down—we give hugs, we put an arm around their shoulder. Touch provides not only physical comfort, but emotional comfort as well, which makes massage such a powerful—and easy to use—tool for relief of tension and stress.

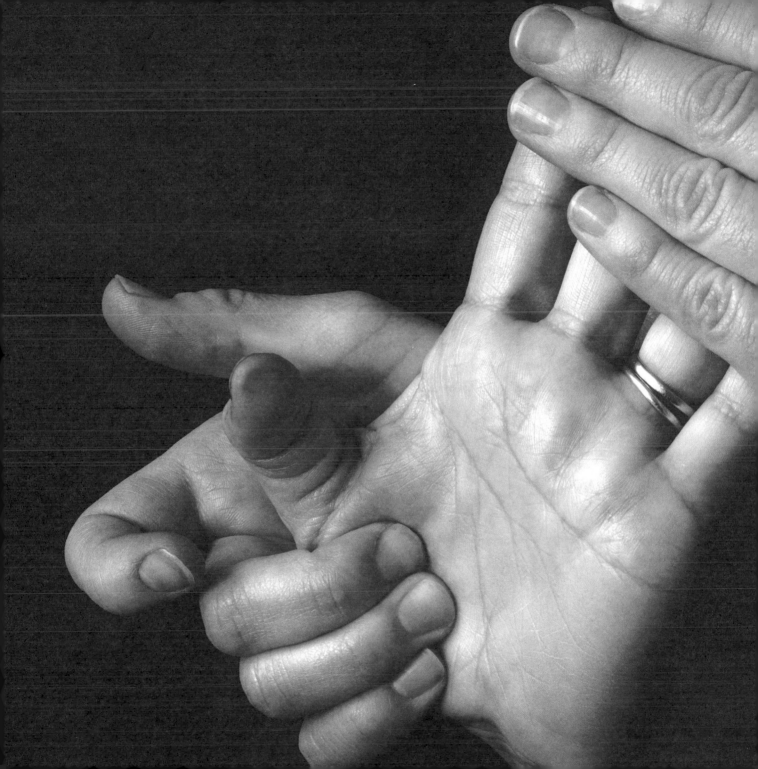

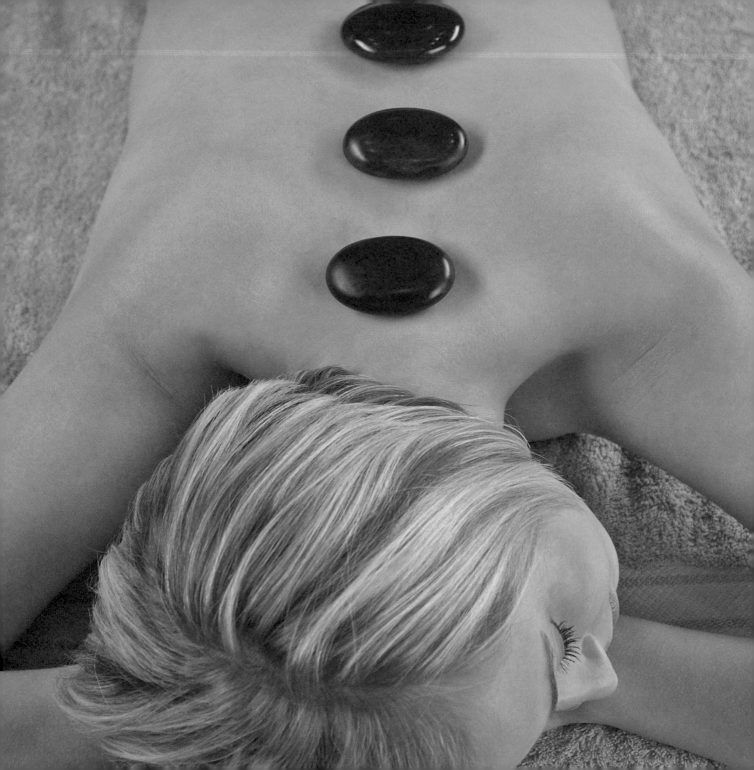

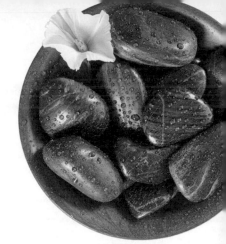

Chapter 1:

It's Getting Hot in Here

The first massage I ever had was a hot stone massage, and it was an extraordinary introduction to the world of massage. Hot stone massage is a unique variant of massage therapy that uses heated stones as part of the massage in order to release tension from the body and calm the nervous system. It is a type of massage that has been practiced for many years and by many cultures, including the Mayan, Native Americans, and Hawaiians, who call it *lomilomi*. *Ayurveda*, an ancient Indian healing tradition, details a universal source of life that affects everything, which is called "prana." In meditation and healing rituals, the hands were used to heal, but also other implements believed to be imbued with this life force, including stones and crystals. Stones from riverbeds were warmed and placed along the energy centers of the body to relax muscles and "extract" tension and pain from the body. The stones were believed to balance and ground the body, harmonizing the essential connection between the mind and the body. The heat and the weight of the stones also mentally and physically focus the body on the massage, allowing the recipient to be more present and receptive.

More recently, the practice of hot stone massage was re-popularized in the United States by an Arizona massage therapist, Mary Nelson, who developed her hot stone massage technique, called LaStone Therapy, in 1994. From then on, its use became more widespread, and hot stone massage is now a staple on the massage menu of most spas. Stones have even been incorporated into other types of massage therapy, including reflexology, facials and pedicures, and sports massage.

The hot stones are placed on certain key points on the body, as well as used as an extension of the massage therapist's hands—not as a replacement. The heat in the stones also allows the massage therapist to work the muscles more deeply without some of the discomfort that is sometimes associated with deep tissue massage—and as a side benefit, the massage therapist gets to experience some of the healing properties of the stones as the massage is performed. Because the therapist is often using the stones to work the body's tissues, hot stone massage reduces strain on the hands, wrists, and arms of the therapist, allowing them to work longer and more efficiently. Remember, however, that the flow of energy goes two ways—just as the stones conduct their heat into the body of your partner and into your hands, they can also transfer emotions from you into your partner—do your best to leave any negative feelings at the door and focus your energy positively into treating your partner.

Experience Matters

Training and experience are essential to performing hot stone massage, so whether you're the client or the therapist, make sure you know what you're getting into before you start. The American Massage Therapy Association requires that in order to become AMTA certified, the massage therapist must graduate from a minimum 500 in-class-hour massage therapy training program, or pass the National Certification Examination in Therapeutic Massage and Bodywork, or possess a current AMTA-accepted license to practice, earn continuing education credit, and uphold the AMTA Code of Ethics.

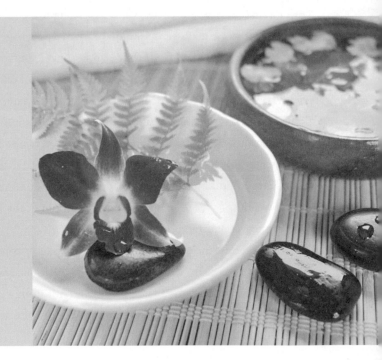

THE FAMILY STONE

What sets hot stone massage apart from other types of massage therapy is the use of smooth, flat stones that are heated in water. The stones used in spas are typically basalt, which retains heat well because it is rich in iron. River rocks are sometimes used because they have been worn smooth by the river. The stones range in size from larger stones for the back, to stones small enough to fit between the toes. The stones are immersed in water and heated until they reach a certain temperature range. Stones are placed on specific points on the body and occasionally on the face, and the massage therapist uses the stones themselves to massage the body.

Basalt stones are often used for hot stone massage, but other kinds of stones can be used as well, as long as they are smooth (in particular, no cracks or sharp edges) and hold heat well. The Internet is a great resource for finding stones. If you're looking for a more natural and inexpensive source of stones, simply troll local beaches or riverbeds for smooth stones of different sizes. Note that some practitioners of hot stone massage believe that in order for the stones to have their maximal effect, naturally smoothed stones, such as those found in rivers or the ocean, must be used because they are intimately connected with the earth—if the stone is mechanically tumbled or polished, it loses some of its healing ability.

Practitioners of hot stone massage believe that different kinds of stones impart different healing effects on the body. Each kind of stone is intricately linked to the earth and to the forces in the earth that created and shaped it. The weight, texture, and even color of the stone used during the massage gives your partner a unique experience and balances the different elements in the body. Pumice, for example, is formed from the separation of gas from lava and is lightweight and porous (all the solidified gas bubbles inside even allow some pumice stones to float). The slightly more abrasive texture imparts a stimulating effect on the body. Stones found on the ocean's shores are typically denser and smoother, as are stones found in riverbeds, though the mineral composition of these rocks differs.

Basalt stones are commonly used for stones that are placed on the body and left to rest for a few minutes. They're also typically used when performing gliding strokes, as their silky surface moves easily over the body. Stones with a bit more texture and an elongated shape, such as some stones found on the coast of New England, work well for edging strokes. The texture should feel somewhat like velvet, not rough or sandpaper-y. As a benefit to the massage therapist, stones with more textured surfaces are easier to hold onto during the massage. You'll read more about the specific strokes later.

The color of the stone also has different results on the body. Black stones, such as basalt, are said to soothe all the elements in the body because black is a combination of all other colors. Stones tinged with green (due to oxidized deposits of copper sulfide within the stone) can alleviate imbalances in the body. Stones with a blue hue have a cooling effect. Blue-gray stones impart peacefulness and extract anger. Some stones have thin stripes of deep red or orange color through them. Light pink stones, such as a rose quartz, can relieve the body of fatigue and heaviness and ease sadness.

Another property of the stones that is essential to their usefulness for a hot stone massage is their ability to retain warmth. Different stones hold heat for varying lengths of time and also radiate heat at different strengths. Igneous, metamorphic, and sedimentary stones typically hold heat well and release it slowly and steadily, making them good for use in massage. Basalt stones, although favored for their silkiness, tend get very hot and give off their heat quickly and unpredictably because they are born of volcanoes, making them more likely to become too hot and burn your partner. However, their origin also imbues basalt stones with great stimulating qualities that will leave the body feeling rejuvenated after a massage. Generally, the darker the color of the stone the hotter it will get and the longer it will remain hot. Using a mixture of types and colors of stones during the massage will expose your partner to a range of healing possibilities.

Shape can also be considered when selecting stones for a massage. Some massage therapists believe that using stones that mirror in shape the part of the body they are placed on increases their ability to heal. For example, a stone placed on the heart chakra would be heart shaped, one for the sacral chakra would resemble the sacral bone, and stones placed on particular muscles would match the shape of those muscles.

In addition, the mineral composition of the stones can also affect the body. Nearly all minerals have some amount of magnetic property. Naturally the stones then, when used on the body, have the potential to act like a magnet—pulling impurities from the body and drawing out stress and negative emotions. Their magnetism can also realign the body's energy and balance the yin and yang forces.

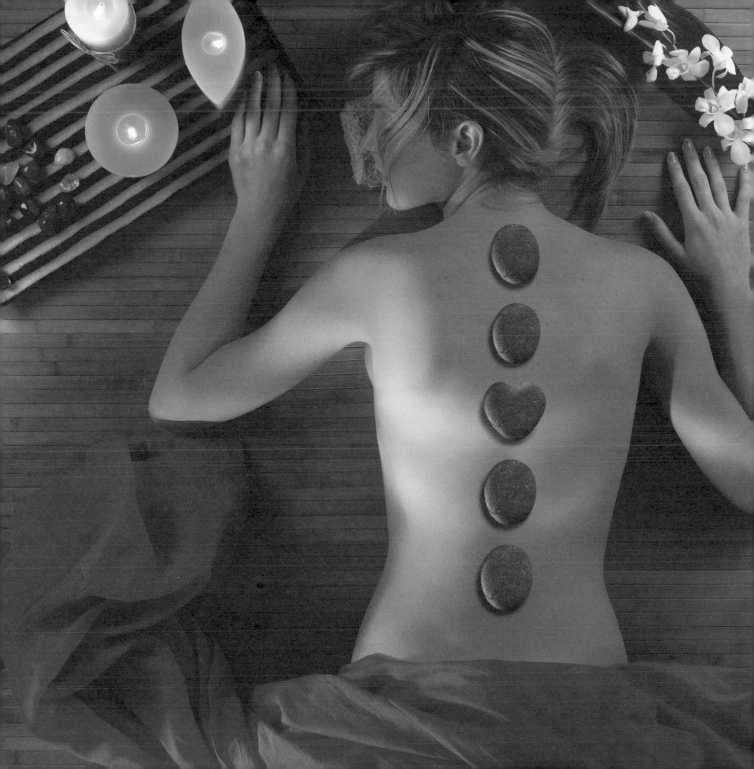

WHERE SOUL MEETS BODY

Chakras are the body's energy centers. It is believed that the chakras act as portals, allowing energy to course in and out of the body's aura. Their purpose is to vitalize the body and help bring a person to self-consciousness. Stones or crystals that correspond to each chakra center are sometimes used during stone massage to stimulate the chakra points, encouraging energy flow throughout the body and grounding it to the earth, providing deep relaxation and stress relief. Moreover, the physical weight of the stones and that they are created and shaped by the earth help ground the person receiving the massage, reconnecting them with the earth.

There are seven major chakras:

1. **Root:** Located at the base of the spine, this is the chakra that keeps the body grounded and connects us to the earth. It is associated with the color red.

2. **Sacral:** Located in the lower abdomen, the sacral chakra is related to our emotions, creativity, and sexuality. It is associated with the color orange.

3. **Solar Plexus:** Located in the solar plexus (a complex network of nerves in the lower abdomen; also called the celiac plexus), this chakra is associated with self-esteem, intuition, and ego. Its color is yellow.

4. **Heart:** Located in the chest, the heart chakra is related to compassion, love, and well-being. The heart chakra can be easily wounded by grief or other emotional trials, but it also has a great capacity for healing. Its color is green or pink.

5. **Throat:** Located in the throat/neck region, the throat chakra is related to communication and self-expression. Speaking honestly and truthfully is the challenge of this chakra. Its color is blue.

6. **Brow (Third Eye):** Located in the center of the forehead, the brow chakra is the portal for wisdom and also regulates our sense of time and awareness of light. The more "open" this chakra is, the more we are able to learn from our experiences and put them in perspective. Its color is indigo.

7. **Crown:** The crown chakra is located above the head, outside of the body. This chakra is called the chakra of consciousness and is responsible for regulating the other chakras. The purpose of the crown chakra is to connect the mind and the body, integrating the whole body. Its color is violet or white.

Specific crystals are sometimes placed on the chakras during hot stone massage to help open them—the crystals are typically not heated or used to massage the body. Although precious gems like sapphires and diamonds do have healing properties, the following stones are more affordable and easy to find. These are just a sampling of the stones associated with each chakra—through further research and hands-on experience you'll discover which stones work best for you and for the person receiving the massage.

Brow (Third-Eye): Amethyst heightens the senses and increases intuition.

Smokey quartz is relaxing and soothes pain; also increases tolerance to stress.

Throat: Moonstones are calming and composing.

Lapis lazuli quiets idle chatter.

Heart: Jade calms irritability; encourages balance and tranquility.

Rose quartz is stress relieving, increases sensitivity and empathy, and opens the heart to self-love and loving others.

Solar Plexus: Citrine placed on the solar plexus can boost self-confidence.

Sacral: Bloodstone promotes creativity and intuition.

Root: Garnet fortifies the inner self and personal strength.

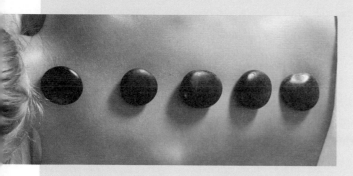

Aura

The colors listed in relation to their chakras are associated with one's aura. An aura is a "halo" of multicolored radiation that surrounds a person and reflects the thoughts or mood of that person.

Another way that hot stone massage can sync up the body and the mind is through the body's meridians. Hot stone massage helps open up these invisible energy pathways that allow *chi* to flow through the body. According to Chinese medicine, chi regulates spiritual, emotional, mental, and physical balance, but it's affected by the opposing forces of yin and yang. When yin and yang are balanced, they have a complementary relationship and keep the body in good health. However, if the flow is interrupted or blocked by anything from environmental pollutants to stress, it creates an imbalance in the body. The 14 meridians (central, governing, circulation/sex, bladder, gallbladder, heart, kidney, large intestine, liver, lung, small intestine, spleen, stomach, and triple warmer) are connected to the body's organ systems, and the goal of ancient healing rituals from acupuncture, herbal therapy, and massage is to restore this balance of chi in the body to keep it functioning at its peak. Hot stone massage restores equilibrium to the body by stimulating specific points connected to the meridians in order to counteract imbalances.

LIVE AND LET GO

The lymphatic system is the body's way of filtering impurities—if you're sick, you may have noticed that your lymph nodes swell—this can be particularly noticeable under your arms or on the sides of your neck under the jaw—because they are filtering more than the usual amount of impurities, working hard to cleanse your system of the illness that has invaded it. A massage goes a long way toward stimulating the lymph system and helping move out impurities to detoxify the body. Moreover, the massage can actually boost the immune system, making your body better prepared to stave off the next attack.

The lymphatic system includes organs, lymph nodes, and vessels—the vessels transport lymph throughout the body, which acts as a kind of garbage collector, picking up dead cells and other waste products, as well as bacteria and viruses. If you're sick or overly stressed, this system bears the brunt of the burden and can slow down, making the body susceptible. Obviously, the lymphatic system plays a key role in your body's overall well-being, so the fact that it can benefit from massage is just one more reason your body deserves one.

If one of the goals of your massage is to stimulate the lymphatic system, let your massage therapist know. They will adjust the speed, direction, and depth of their strokes to maximize their effect on the system. The therapist will also focus the body work on the upper body, including the arms, chest, and face.

The following are some additional conditions that can be alleviated through hot stone massage:

- Muscular aches and pains
- Back pain
- Arthritis
- Fibromyalgia
- Stress and anxiety
- Circulatory problems
- Insomnia
- Depression

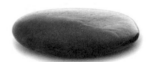

Note that massage therapy should never be considered the only treatment option for any ailment and should be used as part of complete treatment regimen as prescribed by your health professional.

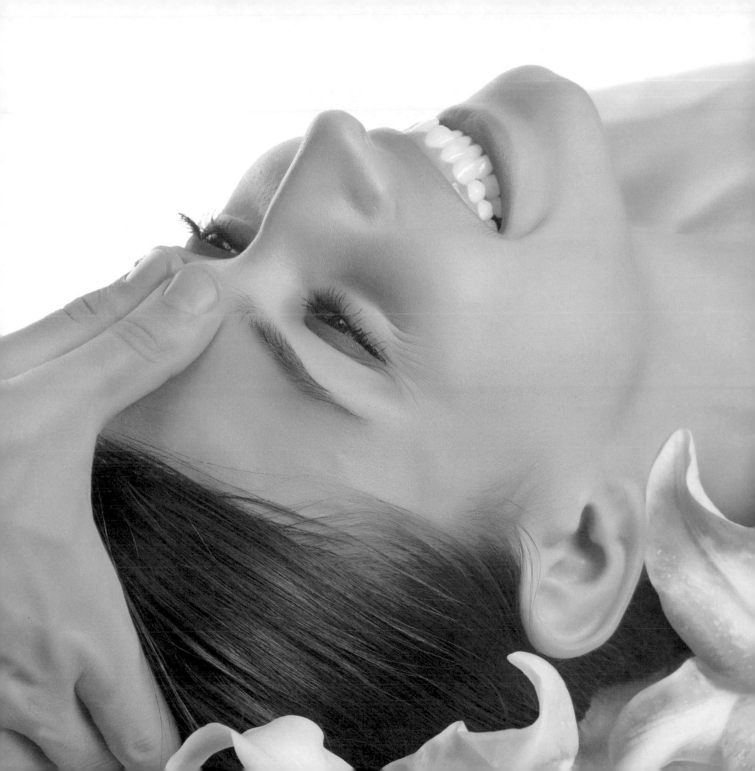

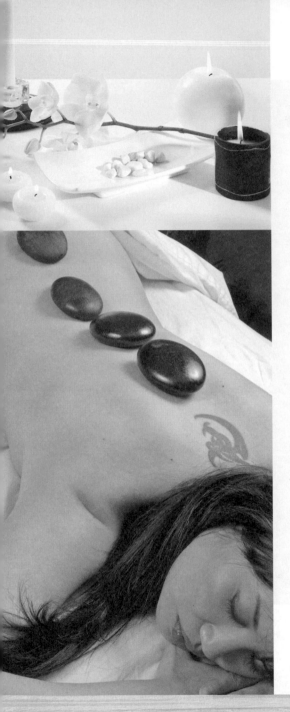

Stone Cold

Stone massage is sometimes also performed using cold stones, which is a form of *cryotherapy* (as opposed to a form of *thermotherapy*, when massage is performed using hot stones). Typically, cooled marble or white quartzite stones are used. The cool temperature of the stones causes the blood vessels to constrict, which can soothe muscle injuries and calm inflammation. Other benefits of using cool stones:

- Refreshing and stimulating to the mind and body
- Can relieve tissue congestion, such as sinus congestion
- Soothes irritation
- Cools down the body's temperature on a hot day or during hot flashes

The cold stones can be particularly effective when placed on the face because this is an area that responds well to the cold for many people. Generally, cold stone massage should be avoided in colder climates and should not be used simultaneously with hot stone massage (a hot stone in one hand and a cold stone in the other) because this can be jarring to your partner, counteracting the relaxing effects of the stones.

The following are few techniques that are well suited for cold stone massage:

- **Cocooning** involves surrounding a specific body part with cold stones to soothe muscle and joint inflammation. (This technique can also be used with warm stones, as you'll read later.) Cocoons are placed at the beginning of the session and removed about half-way (approximately 10 minutes) through.

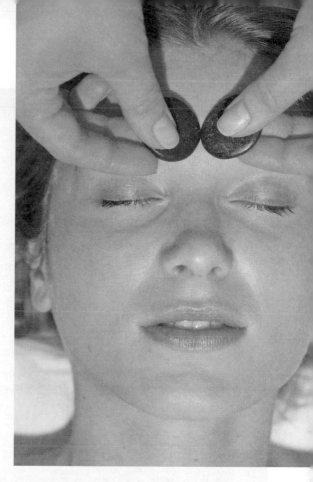

- **Thermal contrasting** is when your partner is massaged with gliding strokes, alternating hot and cold stones on the skin. The back and forth between the extremes of temperatures causes the blood vessels to expand and constrict, stimulating the movement of impurities out of the body and leaving the skin firm and glowing and the body reawakened. Also, performing this technique on the belly can relieve stagnation or constipation.
- **Cryofacial balancing** focuses on the face and uses cold stones, stroked smoothly over the face, to cool and quiet skin that has been inflamed or irritated by a waxing or peel.
- **Eye balancing** uses small, flat, cold stones laid on the eyes to calm red, swollen eyes.

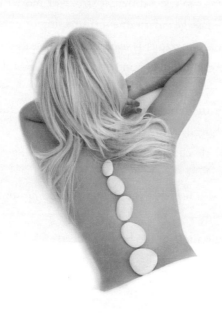

Before, During, and After the Massage

The following tips will help you make the most of your massage experience.

• Be open and receptive to the potential healing benefits of the massage.

• Try not to eat just before your massage.

• Arrive on time so you can fill out any necessary paperwork, but also so you can start to mentally relax and prepare for your massage.

• During the massage, if you are not comfortable removing your clothes entirely, wear clothing that won't constrict you and which will allow the massage therapist to work the parts of the body in need of a massage. Remove bulky jewelry that might interfere with the massage.

• If you have any health conditions that could be impacted, by having a massage, be sure to give the massage therapist a full, accurate report.

• Communication with the massage therapist is essential. Talk with the therapist before you start about any particular areas you'd like them to focus on. During the massage, if anything the therapist is doing is painful or uncomfortable, be sure to speak up. If you'd like the therapist to use a different stroke or more pressure, also let them know. Moreover, if you find anything about the massage environment distracting or unpleasant (music, the scent of a candle, the level of light, or if your massage therapist is overly chatty), speak up.

• Remember to breathe throughout the massage. Steady breathing will help the body and mind relax and absorb the effects of the massage.

• Try to relax your muscles as much as possible. Contracting, or tightening, the muscles (which you might do if you're nervous or if a sensitive area of the body is being massaged) counteracts the effects of the massage.

• Relaxing the mind is equally important. If you're having trouble clearing your mind, try focusing on your breath or on the rhythmic strokes of the massage.

• If you're not happy with the way the massage is going, or if you feel that the therapist is doing something inappropriate, you have the right to stop the massage at any time.

• Take time to be calm and still after your massage. This will help prolong the healing effects.

Although massage therapy should be indulged in as often as possible to maximize its benefits, the reality of our hectic lives is that time to relax must often be scheduled in, and when time is at a premium, taking time for ourselves is often the first thing to go. A few tips on how to make the most of your time with your massage therapist after the session is complete:

- Drink water post-massage. During a massage, just like when you exercise, toxins are flushed from the system. Drinking water after your massage aids in and speeds up this process.

- Stretching between massage sessions helps maintain the muscle relaxation gained during your massage. Stretching can be in the form or yoga or just a regular stretching routine, and need only be 5 or 10 minutes daily.

- Taking care of your body in general supports the effects of massage—this means regular exercise, a healthy diet, and being aware of the needs of your body—getting extra rest when you need it and not consistently pushing your body to its limits.

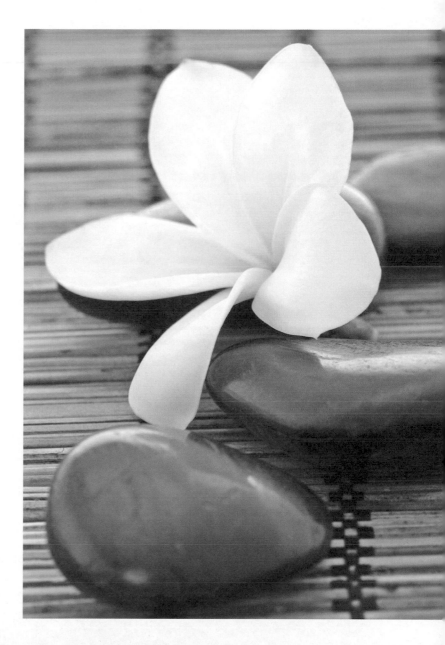

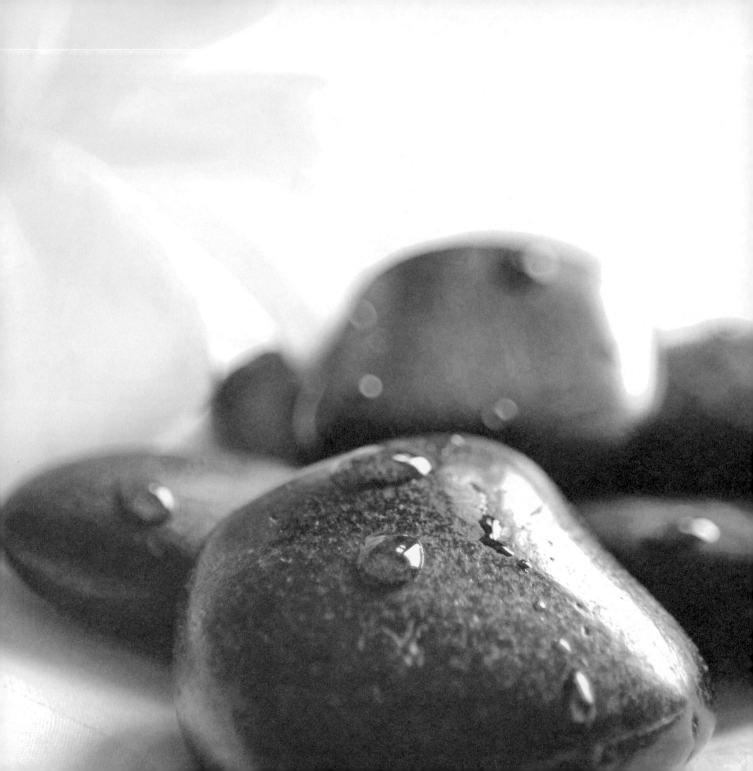

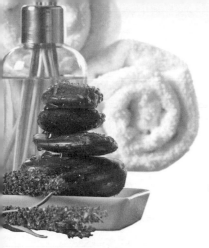

CHAPTER 2:

GETTING STARTED: THE HOT STONE MASSAGE

Now that you know some of the basics, it's time for the massage itself. If you're giving or receiving a hot stone massage, you can expect the following items to be part of the process:

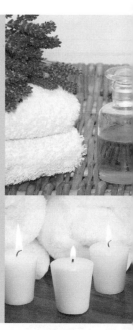

- Stones
- Massage oil
- Massage table
- Linens for the table
- Towels or a flannel blanket to drape the massage recipient
- A heating unit for the stones and tongs or a slotted spoon to remove the stones from the water. (Note: if the heating unit does not have a temperature gauge, you'll need a kitchen thermometer to measure the water's temperature.) There are heating units created especially for hot stone massage available, but you can use anything from a crock pot to a large bowl of hot water.
- Optional: candles or soft music. Some people think these items add to the overall experience by incorporating all of the body's senses, but some find them to be a distraction. Check with your partner as to their preference.

If you're limited for time or space, you can isolate the massage to a particularly stressed area, such as the feet, hands, or shoulders. See Appendix A (pages 47-53) on basic massage strokes for tips on working these individual areas.

You'll need around 40 or 50 stones of varying sizes to give a hot stone massage—fewer stones can be used, but they'll need to be reheated more often. The stones typically take 10 minutes or more to heat up, so make sure to start the heating process in advance.

Similar to when a patient sees their doctor, the massage recipient is putting themselves in vulnerable position and trusting the massage therapist with their body. Everything possible must be done to retain this trust—including keeping clean and sanitary stones and workplace. Stones should be cleaned using hot soapy water between each session and the water heating the rocks should be changed. At the end of each day, stones should be sanitized.

Read ahead to the section on aromatherapy for a review of incorporating essential oils into the massage, as well as a few sample oil blends.

Giving the Massage

Now that the massage area is set up and your partner is mentally and physically ready for the treatment, you can begin the massage.

Monitor the temperature of the water, heating stones closely throughout the massage. It should be around 110 or 120 degrees Fahrenheit, and never hotter than 130 degrees Fahrenheit or you risk burning your massage partner. If the stones are too hot to handle, it's likely they'll be uncomfortable for the person who is receiving the massage as well. Be sure to ask how the stones feel and keep up this dialogue throughout the massage; likewise, if you're getting the massage, be sure to speak up if the stones are too hot for you—you'll never get the full benefit of the treatment if you're wincing in pain the entire time.

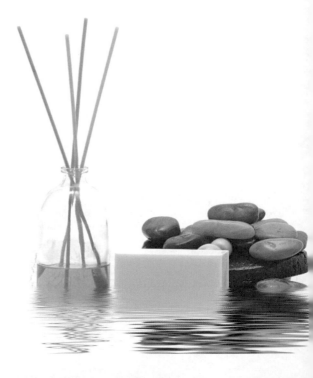

Note that there is some disagreement in the massage community about whether stones should placed directly on the skin and left to rest. Some argue that the body cannot experience the full healing power of the stones unless they are placed directly on the skin, whereas others feel that a protective barrier, such as a flannel sheet or thick towel, should always come between the skin and the stone. Discuss with your partner before you begin the massage about which option is preferable to him or her.

SAMPLE MASSAGE I

As you perform the massage, keep in mind that certain areas of the body, such as the face, elbows, and behind the knees can be more sensitive, so adjust your pressure and stroke and check in with the client when massaging these areas.

The following are some strokes that work particularly well with hot stone massage. Refer to Appendix A (pages 47-53) on basic massage strokes for some additional strokes.

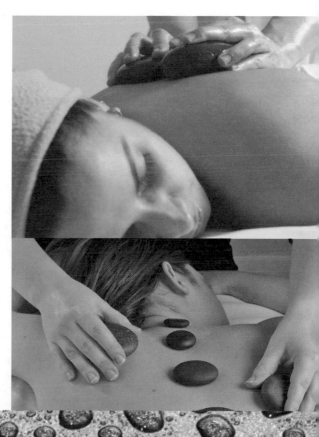

- **Gliding** is the basic hot stone massage stroke. For this stroke, the flat side of the stone is used to massage the body in long strokes, using moderate to strong pressure. Make sure to keep the body well oiled when using this stroke. Try to think of the stones merely as an extension of your hand when performing this stroke rather than as a tool.
- **Edging** is a technique that will work the tissue more deeply. It is performed using the side of the stone rather than the flat surface. Hold the stone with your thumb on one side and the rest of your fingers lightly gripping the other side, as if you were pinching the stone. Use a deeper level of pressure and slow strokes to work the tissue in the direction of the muscle fibers.
- **Flushing** is a stroke that is similar to gliding and can be used following the edging stroke. This is a cleansing stroke that

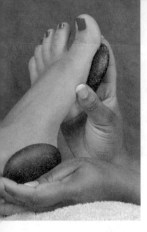

helps the body work out some of the toxins released during the massage. Flushing should be performed in the direction of one of the terminal points on the body, so the impurities are able to exit the body—according to Ayurveda, these are the crown of the head, ears, genitals, hands, and the soles of the feet.

- **Cocooning** is a hot stone technique that can be used to treat a localized area. If a certain part of the body is particularly stiff, a "cocoon" of heated stones are placed around the area at the beginning of the massage and removed at the midpoint of the session.

In addition to the strokes used during the massage, as you place stones on the body and remove them and as you move to another part of the body, the physically lifting off of the stones helps imbue the body with a sense of lightness or weightlessness throughout the massage.

Note: Whenever you are transferring stones from the heating unit to the body, make sure you stand to the side of the massage table where you are placing the stones. Stones can become slippery, especially with the addition of massage oil—never move a stone across the face area. Nothing would disrupt the serenity of the massage like a dropped stone!

Prepare the massage table or area you're using with clean linens. Start with your partner laying on his or her back, draped with towels or a blanket. Begin the massage by selecting eight

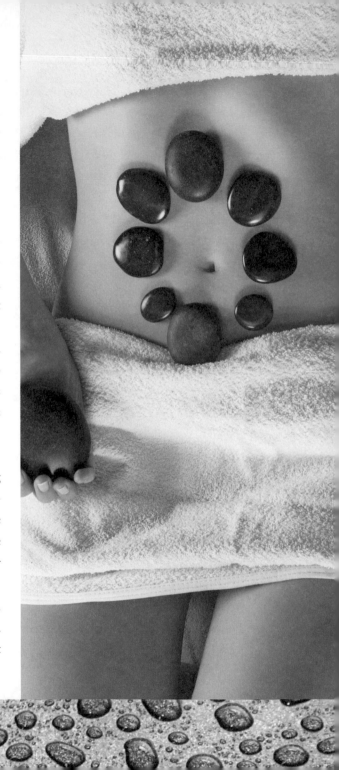

smaller stones and placing them between the client's toes. Wrap the feet firmly with a towel. Next place a larger stone on each thigh. Place a medium-sized stone in the palm of each hand.

Move to the upper part of the body, and place a large stone beneath each shoulder, between the spine and the shoulder blade. You can then place a line of smaller stones down the breastbone and a larger stone on each chest muscle.

The head is next. Use four smaller stones, placing one underneath the lips on the chin, one on each cheek, and one on the forehead (the brow, or third eye, chakra discussed earlier).

Remember to periodically check in on your partner's comfort with the stones' heat and, once you begin massaging the muscles, be sure to ask if your level of pressure is comfortable—sometimes the client may want a little more or a little less. Also, check the temperature for any stones that you leave resting on the body—if they begin to feel cool, replace them with fresh hot stones.

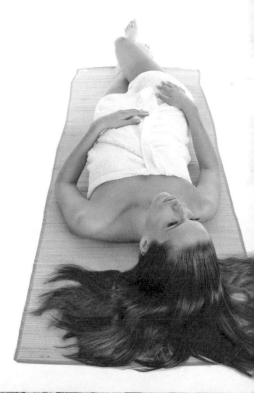

Return to the feet and remove the stones, placing them back in the hot water. Select your massage oil, undrape one leg, and apply it to the feet and calf area. (It's best to keep any portions of the body draped that are not being worked—this enhances the comfort of your partner and also helps retain the warmth of the stones.) Use a smaller stone to massage the foot from the top of the foot and ankle to the heel and arch of the foot. Remove the stones resting on the thighs, select a medium-sized stone, and massage the shin and thigh, moving from the extremities toward the trunk of the body. Drape the leg you massaged and repeat on the other leg.

Effleurage (from the French word *effleurer*, meaning "to skim over") is one of the most commonly used massage techniques, consisting of long, slow, gliding strokes, performed with open hands. Typically, effleurage is the first type of stroking during the massage because it has a calming effect. Effleurage is usually performed in the direction of the heart to promote circulation and lymphatic drainage.

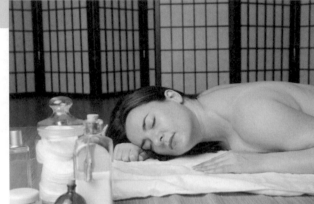

Move on to the arms next. Except for the palms, stones are difficult to balance on the arms, so they are usually just massaged. Undrape one arm and apply massage oil. As with the feet, use a smaller stone to massage the hand and wrist. Use a medium stone to massage the forearm and upper arm. Cover the arm and repeat on the other arm.

Remove the stones from the chest and from the face. Gently massage the face (no massage oil is needed for the face), using a circular motion over the cheeks and forehead combined with light strokes. Next, massage the scalp as if you were giving a shampoo. You can also work the neck and shoulder regions at this time.

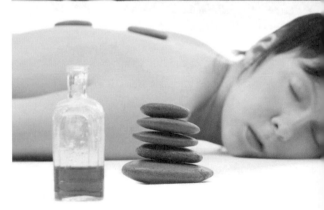

Remove any remaining stones, and now have your partner turn over. Make it easier by discreetly lifting the towel or blanket, allowing him or her to flip onto their stomach. Line the back of the legs with fresh stones. Put a large stone on the bottom of each foot, wrapping each with a towel to hold it in place. Place stones along the spine and cover the back. Massage the backs of the legs and the back as you did the front.

Allow your partner to rest for a few minutes after the massage and soak in the soothing effects.

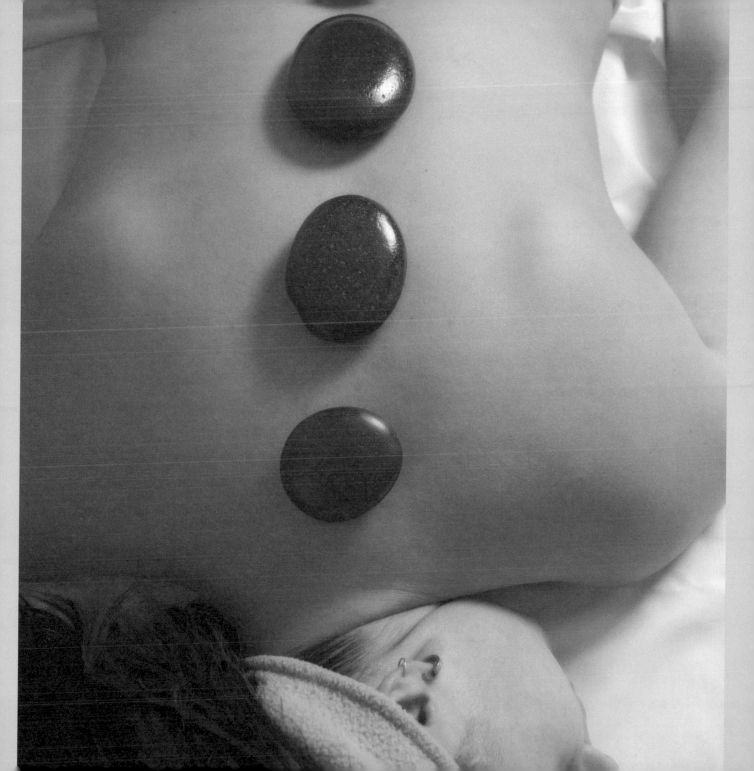

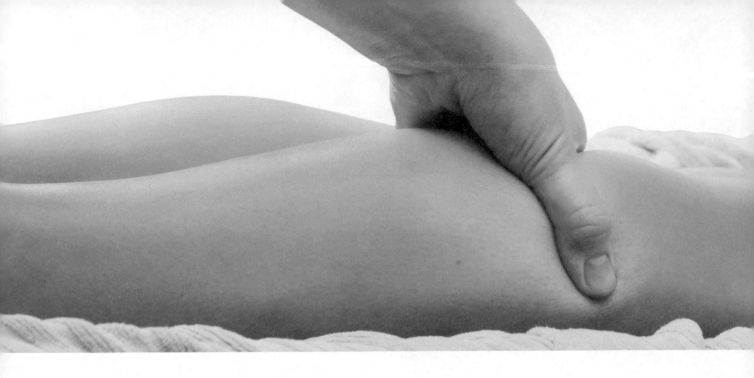

SAMPLE MASSAGE 2

Follow the tips for setting up and performing the massage, as well as the precautions listed for the first sample massage. This massage is slightly shorter and less involved than the first massage.

Your partner should start lying on his or her stomach. Undrape one leg and place a hot stone on the upper leg, middle of the hamstring, back of the knee, and on the center of the calf.

Massage the leg using the appropriate stroke for the type of massage desired by your partner, making sure to glide the stones in the direction of the heart. Next, move the stones from the leg you just worked to the opposite leg (replacing them with fresh stones if they have cooled). Redrape the first leg. Massage the second leg. Take the stones off the second leg and cover both legs.

On top of the drape covering the back, make a small pile of stones on the lower back to warm up the muscles. If your partner is comfortable with this, you can now massage the glutes.

The back will be worked next. Place stones on the shoulders and on the back of the neck. Remove the pile of stones from the lower back and massage this part of the back.

Next, remove the stones from the upper back area and massage here. Note how each part of the body is being warmed by the resting stones before being worked by massage strokes. Have your partner flip onto his or her back.

Again, start with the legs. Place stones on the top, middle, and lower thigh of both legs. Drape both legs and place stones on the upper, mid, and low thigh of both legs. Place smaller stones between the toes, securing them in place as necessary. Allow the legs to heat up, and move to the arms. Stones can be tricky to keep steady on the arms, so simply massage them with steady, smooth strokes.

Next, place stones on the upper chest area. Return to the legs and remove the stones from one leg at a time and massage the front the leg. Repeat on the other leg.

If your partner wants you to massage the abdomen be sure to stroke in a counterclockwise direction in order to follow the intestinal tract.

Take the stones off the upper chest and massage this area, as well as the neck. Complete the massage with a gentle face and scalp massage. Although you can rest stones on the face if your partner wishes, the face and scalp can be sensitive, so stones are typically not used for massaging these areas.

See Appendix A (pages 47-53) on basic massage techniques for more specific instructions about massaging different parts of the body.

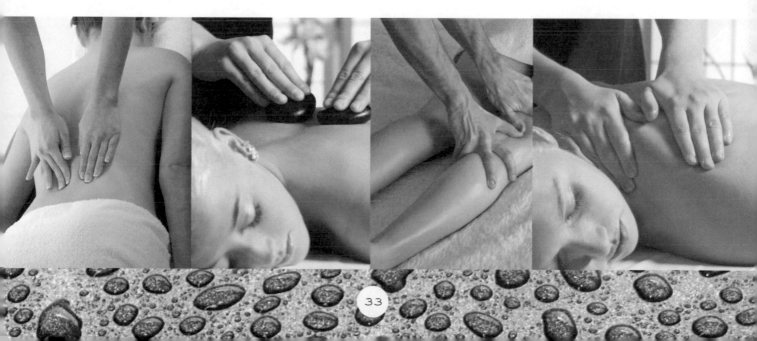

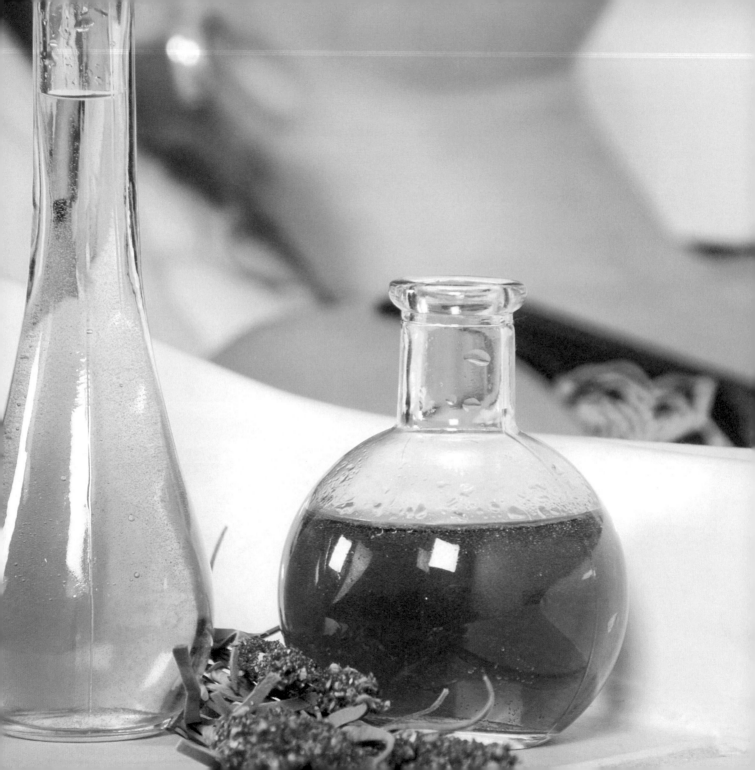

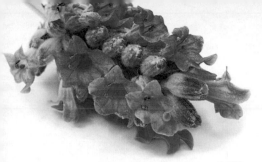

Chapter 3:

Aromatherapy and Massage

Touch has a powerful ability to calm and heal; likewise, our sense of smell can have potent effects on the mind and body. Scent is the only sense that is intricately linked with our memory—a particular scent has an uncanny ability to prompt the recall of past experiences. Have you ever caught a quick whiff of a scent in the air and been blindsided by a memory of an old boyfriend or girlfriend or been transported back to your childhood home? Using scented aromatherapy during massage combines the senses touch and smell to create a fuller, more therapeutic experience. When the nose inhales, it draws in the molecules that something gives off—its scent. These molecules are absorbed by a special patch of neurons at the top of your nasal passages that perceive the smell and transmit it to your brain, triggering a memory or response—synthesizing the mind and the body while simultaneously soothing and refreshing the body's largest organ—the skin.

The practice of aromatherapy can be seen as an offshoot of the Ayurvedic principle of prana, which was discussed earlier. Because this life force surges through everything, it makes sense that flowers, plants, and herbs would have healing and rejuvenating effects on the body. Essential oils are extracted from the plant or flower through a process of distillation, and these concentrated oils are used for many purposes: sometimes for the soothing properties of their scent alone, but also in conjunction with other therapies, such as massage.

There are about 3,000 essential oils in the world, so you can imagine the wide range of conditions that can potentially be treated using essential oils. In combination with massage, the healing properties of the oils come not only from their contact with the skin, but the effects of their aroma, creating a deeper, more effective massage

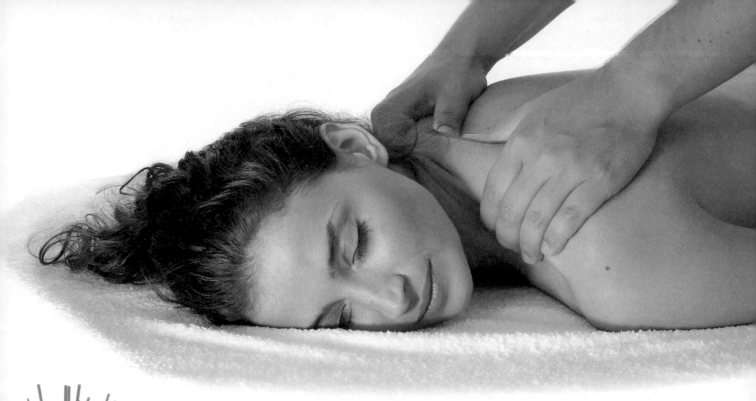

experience. Moreover, when essentials oils are used during a hot stone massage, the warmth generated by the draped body, the hot stones, and the warm hands of the massage therapist speeds the process of absorption of the oils. The stones can also be heated in water that has a few drops of essential oil in it.

Note: Some oils should not be used when pregnant or if you have certain skin conditions. Check with your health professional before using any essential oils.

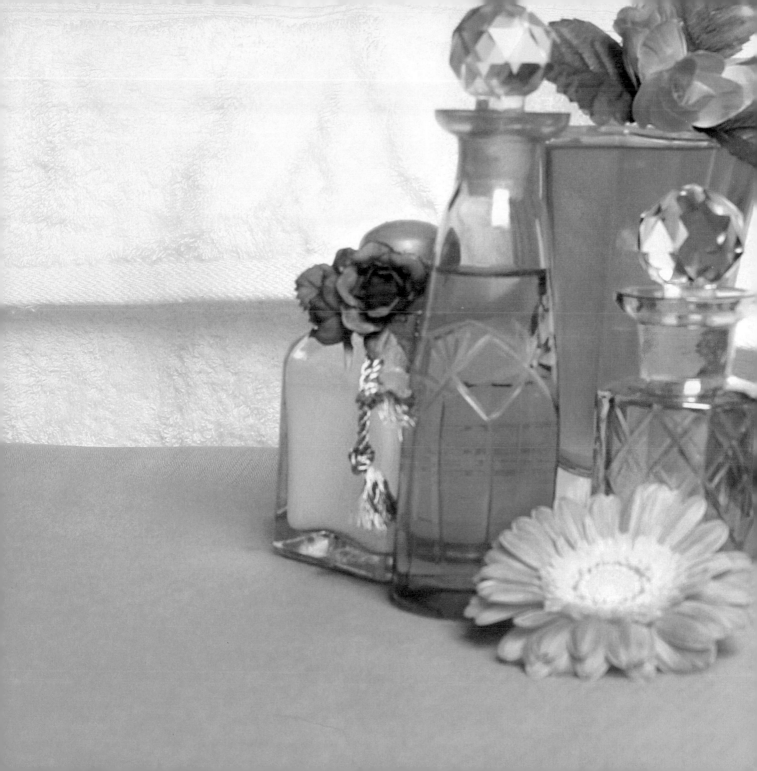

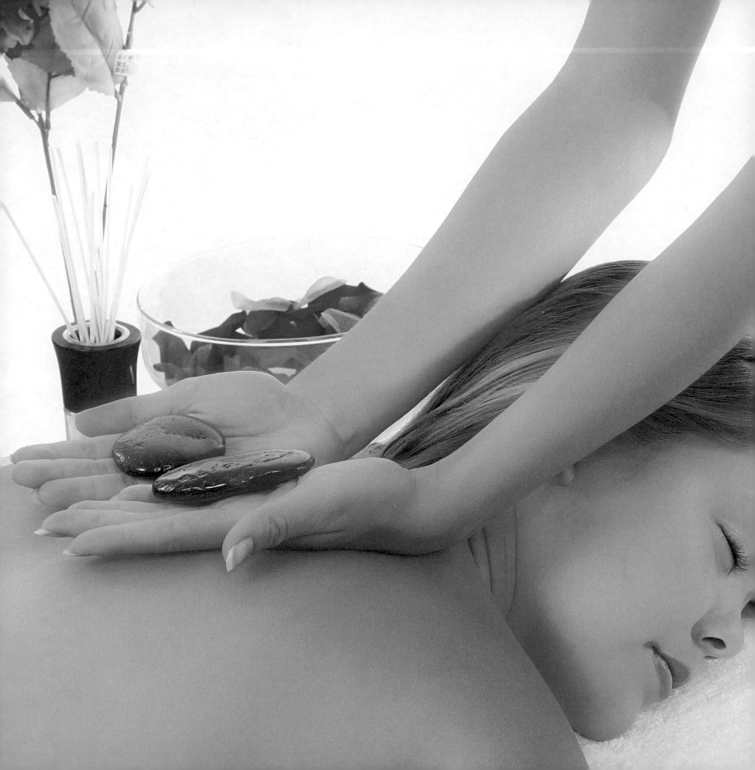

RECIPES

Note: Never apply undiluted oil on the skin without using a base or carrier oil (such as sweet almond oil, hazelnut oil, sunflower oil, or grapeseed oil). Refer to Appendix B (pages 53-55) for a list of oils and their therapeutic effects.

Anxiety:

Lavender, 10 drops

Geranium, 5 drops

Sandalwood, 10 drops

Blend into 2 oz. of the base/carrier oil such as jojoba. Massage into chest, back, and neck.

OR

Lavender, 6 drops

Frankincense, 8 drops

Sandalwood, 6 drops

Blend into 2 oz. of the base/carrier oil such as jojoba. Massage into chest, back, and neck.

Stress:

Bergamot, 10 drops

Frankincense, 8 drops

Rose or jasmine, 2 drops

Blend into 2 oz. of the base/carrier oil and massage into the chest, back, and neck.

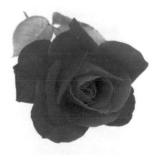

General muscle aches:

Lavender, 2 drops

Rosemary, 2 drops

Add 2 drops lavender and 2 drops rosemary oil to 4 teaspoons of any plain base/carrier oil. Use for a gentle body massage.

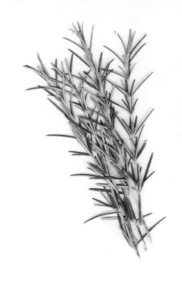

Backache:

Eucalyptus, 2 drops

Lavender, 2 drops

Lemon, 1 drop

Blend into 2 oz. of the base/carrier oil. Massage into the back using the fingertips.

Circulation:

Lavender, 6 drops

Rosemary, 4 drops

Vetiver, 2 drops

Blend into 4 oz. of sesame oil and massage over the body.

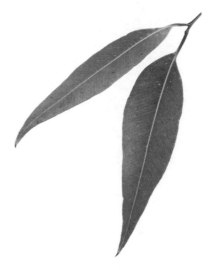

Hands:

Lime, 5 drops

Thyme, 5 drops

Eucalyptus, 5 drops

Cajeput, 5 drops

Blend into 4 tablespoons of the base/carrier oil and massage on the hands.

Legs:

Cypress, 2 drops

Lime, 2 drops

Lemon, 1 drop

Blend into 2 ml. of the base/carrier oil and massage into the calves.

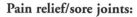

Pain relief/sore joints:

Pine, 3 drops

Eucalyptus, 3 drops

Frankincense, 3 drops

Blend into 20 ml. of the base/carrier oil and massage over the body or a particularly sore area.

Calming/relaxing:

Neroli, 3 drops

Jasmine, 2 drops

Blend into 20 ml. of the base/carrier oil.

Stimulating/uplifting:

Peppermint, 1 drop

Myrrh, 1 drop

Lavender, 2 drops

Blend into 20 ml. of the base/carrier oil.

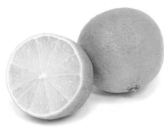

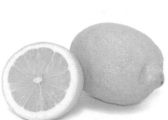

Blend Well

When you first begin incorporating essential oils into your massage, following a set recipe is probably best. Once you're more comfortable with the oils and their properties, you might want to try your hand at blending your own—let the following tips (and your nose) guide you in the right direction.

- Floral: Lavender, jasmine
- Woodsy: Pine, cedar
- Earthy: Vetiver, patchouli
- Herbaceous: Marjoram, rosemary, basil
- Minty: Peppermint
- Medicinal: Eucalyptus, tea tree
- Spicy: Nutmeg, clove, cinnamon
- Citrusy: Orange, lemon, lime

Generally, oils that are in the same scent category mix well with each other. The following categories also complement each other:

- Florals and spicy, citrusy and woodsy oils
- Woodsy oils work well with most other categories
- Spicy oils blend well with florals and citrus oils
- Minty scents blend well with citrus, woodsy, herbaceous and earthy oils

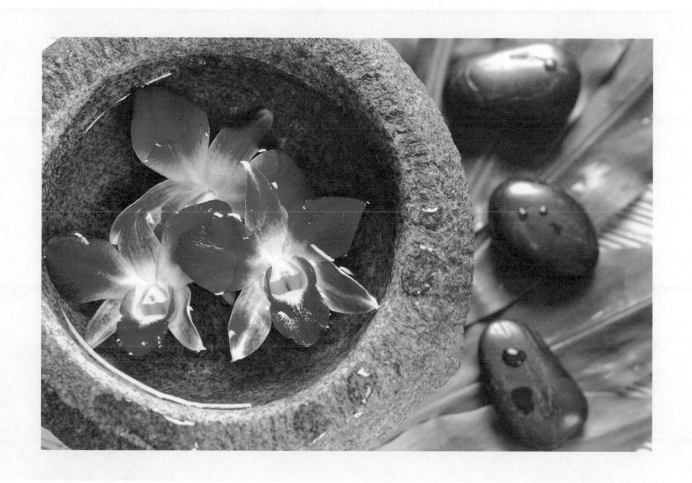

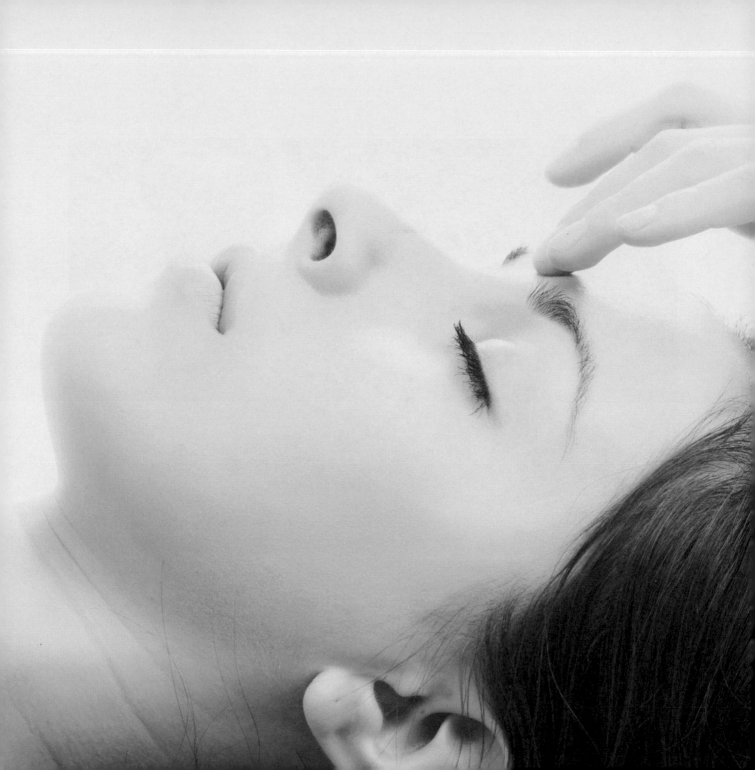

Finishing Strokes

Now that you have all the basic information on how to give (and receive) a hot stone massage, you can begin incorporating massage into your lifestyle. You'll soon notice that you're feeling more balanced—mentally and physically. Hot stone massage is a distinctive experience that will deeply relax your aching and tired muscles and calm the mind. Sometimes it seems like it's just impossible to snag even a few minutes of spare time, but if you take a little time for yourself on a regular basis, you'll be better able to serve your friends, family, and job!

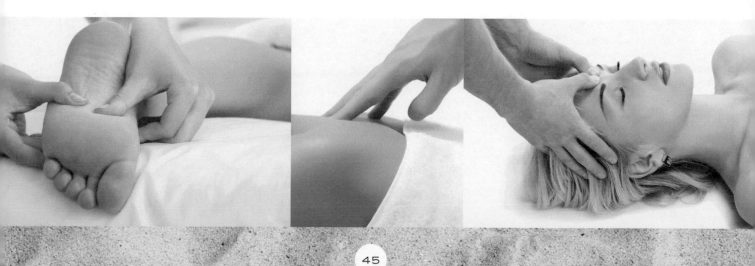

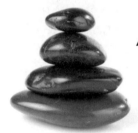 Appendixes

Note: For all of these massages, apply oil as needed to the body to ensure smooth, warm stroking.

Incorporate some of the following basic massage strokes and techniques into your hot stone massage. You'll notice that it can be hard to completely isolate a body part—the back massage overlaps with the neck, the leg massage with the foot, and so on. These tips will get you started, but you'll soon develop your own sense of what works best and seems to benefit your massage partner the most. However, you should always be prepared to adjust your techniques on a case-by-case basis, depending on what the person receiving the massage asks for. Hot stones can be easily incorporated into any of the following methods.

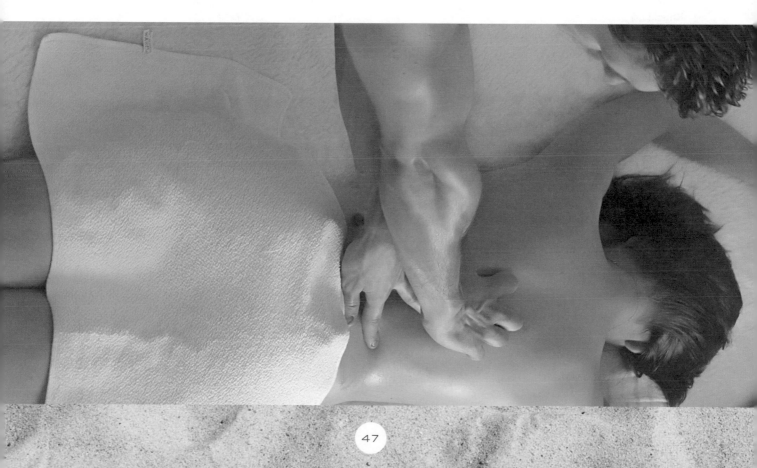

Basic Massage Strokes

Stroking (Effleurage)

This is the easiest and most commonly used massage stroke. It is typically used to begin a massage. Glide your hands over the body, using flat hands and long, rhythmic strokes. This type of movement will relax your massage partner into the massage and prepare the body for deeper massage work.

Kneading (Petrissage)

Petrissage is a category of stroke that covers any stroke that involves squeezing or gripping the muscles, including kneading or wringing. It is most commonly used on thighs, glutes, calves, and shoulders. When using this stroke, grip the muscles firmly and knead and roll them with slow, deep movements, making sure that your hands are working together in a coordinated motion.

Knuckling

Knuckling is a technique most often used on the upper chest and shoulders. Press the knuckles into the area being massaged and use a rotating motion to work the muscles, relieving stress and tension.

Tapping (Tapotement)

Tapotement is a category of strokes that encompasses any "percussive" massage techniques, such as pummeling, hacking, and cupping. In pummeling, you pound (firmly, but never aggressively) the softer areas of the body, such as the glutes and thighs, with loose fists, using the pinky finger side of the hand. This movement eases tension and gets the blood circulating. Hacking is more of a "karate chop" motion, where the body is pounded with a straight, open hand. Cupping is performed by positioning the hand with fingers bent at a 90-degree angle, keeping the fingers straight, and using the hollow part of the fists alternately in rapid up-and-down movements. For these strokes, maintain loose hands and wrists, and try to stroke the body in a fluid, rhythmic manner.

Friction

Friction strokes are designed to work the muscle tissue more deeply and are usually applied later in the massage. The fingers, heels of the palm, and thumbs are used to work the muscles, either fast or slow, generating heat in the muscles and relaxing tight muscles, soothing sore joints, and increasing circulation.

Deep Tissue

Deep tissue techniques are typically used when one wants to work a specific area. By focusing on one problem joint, muscle, or group of muscles, the massage therapist can work deeper layers of the soft tissue. This technique can help relieve chronic stress through slow strokes and deep finger pressure.

Feathering

This light, gentle stroke is usually used at the end of the massage and is done with light, quick strokes using just the fingertips.

NECK AND SHOULDERS

The neck and shoulder area is where many people carry a lot of their stress and tension. If you've ever tried consciously relaxing the muscles in your body, you'll find that most of the time your shoulders and neck are tense and raised, not fully relaxed. The following basic tips will help release the muscle tension in these areas. If just the neck area needs refreshing, this massage can be performed with your partner seated in front of you.

Have your partner lie on his or her back; stand at the top of their head. Knead the tops of the shoulders—because this is an area where many people carry a lot of tension—a fair amount of pressure can be used. Use the tips of the fingers and make small circular motions, starting at the base of the neck and working up toward the head. Alternately, you can also use the thumbs to gently knead the neck, using the same circular motion. Perform a neck massage by positioning your hands as if you were going to grip the neck (it's probably easiest to be standing at the side of the head for this) and rub the neck using both hands so the whole neck is covered, but alternating hands. Repeat about 20 times. Follow with smooth downward strokes from the base of the head to the shoulders. Cover the entire neck area. Follow this by gently squeezing the back of the neck.

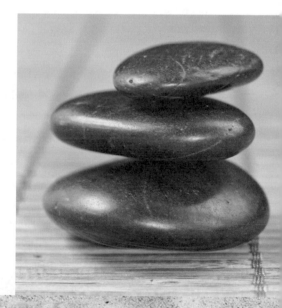

Chest and Abdomen

It's easiest to perform the chest massage, either sitting or standing, positioned at the top of the body.

Start by using your fingertips to stroke between the upper ribs. Next, using a circular motion, massage down the breastbone, following the lines of the ribs out and up the sides of the body. Now, starting from the bottom of the rib cage, use both hands on one side of the chest and stroke upward. Finally, place both your hands on the chest and stroke firmly out toward the shoulders.

Next, move to the abdomen. This is a sensitive area for many people because it is soft and vulnerable. Be sure to check with your partner that it is okay to massage this area, and make sure they are at ease throughout the massage.

Using both hands, softly massage the around the belly button in a counterclockwise direction. Continue this motion, but switch to using your fingertips and make small circles as you stroke. Finally, place a hand on each hip, and stroke upward the length of the torso a few times, then move up and over the breastbone and off the shoulders.

Back

Our backs see a lot of action—whether you're doing heavy lifting or slouched in a chair in front of a computer. The back supports our body all day long. A basic massage that works the upper and lower back will help ease some of the strain on these muscles.

Start at the lower back and use your whole hand (both of them) to stroke the back with long, slow movements. Move straight up the back toward the neck. Next, separate your hands, bring one to each shoulder, gently massaging the shoulder, and sliding your hands back down the back and sides.

Switch from using your whole hand to just the thumbs. Along the spine of the lower back, make short, quick strokes using the balls of your thumbs in the direction of the head. Move to the upper back and continue to use your thumbs to massage the neck area. Gently knead the neck, from the base of the neck to the top, using a circular motion. Then use a smooth, even stroke down the neck toward the shoulders.

Next, move your hands to the middle of the back, change back to using your whole hand, but with your fingers spread, and massage the back up and out in the direction of the shoulders.

Complete the massage by using just your fingertips to lightly stroke the back, from neck to lower back.

Legs

From standing all day in heels to completing a strenuous workout session, the legs are what (literally) keep us going, and they support quite a load. Massaging this area will relieve some of the stress and tension built up over the course of a long day spent on your feet.

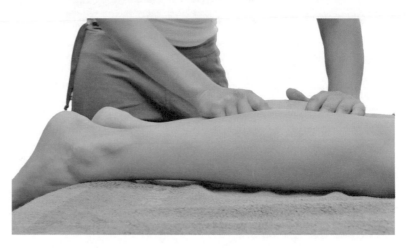

Start with your partner on his or her stomach so you can work the back of the legs. Warm up the leg for massage by covering it with oil, using both hands to make smooth, gentle strokes over the entire leg. Next, knead the thigh and calf by gripping the leg lightly with your hands and using your thumbs to massage the muscles. Finish the massage by massaging the entire leg as if you were wringing out a wet shirt, with each hand moving in the opposite direction over the leg. Finally, stroke the leg lightly with your fingertips. Remember to be mindful of the sensitive area at the back of the knee. Cover the leg and perform the massage on the opposite leg.

To massage the front of the leg, your partner should lie on his or her back. When performing a full body massage, you might consider massaging the tops of the legs after massaging the feet. Place both hands on either side of the calf, just above the ankle. Stroke up the leg, using long, smooth strokes. Apply a bit more pressure using firm strokes as you move up the leg and massage around the hip area. Lighten your strokes as you move back down the leg and along the sides of the legs. Next, as with the back of the leg, massage the entire leg with a circular kneading motion.

Massage the upper thigh. If you're working the right leg, stand on the left side of the body to do this and vice versa. Knead the area as you did the front of the leg, lightly gripping the thigh and kneading with the thumbs over the entire thigh. Lift the muscle of the thigh slightly as you do this. Repeat the "wringing" technique you used on the back of the leg on the front of the leg. If you're standing on the right side of the body, the palms of your hands should be close to your body and your fingers on the inside of the leg as you move the hands in opposite directions, "wringing" the leg. Start at the ankle and move up the leg.

Hands and Feet

Our hands and feet are what carry us through the day and do most of our work for us. Use the following techniques to give them a soothing, recuperative massage.

Let's start with the feet. Start by massaging the top of the foot, moving in from the toes to the ankle. Next, stroke the bottom of the foot, increasing your pressure as you work. Remember that many people's feet are sensitive, so be mindful of the person's reactions as you work.

Next, use a circular stroke over the entire foot using your thumbs. You can increase pressure when you work areas like the ball of the foot and the heel because the skin is usually thicker in these areas. Don't forget to massage the sides of the feet, too.

Lift the foot and rotate the ankle in one direction and then the other, about five times in each direction.

Work the sole of the foot again by making your hand into a fist and kneading the bottom of the foot—be mindful of the amount of pressure you use. Pay particular attention to the arch of the foot.

Don't forget the toes! Massage each toe individually by softly rolling it between your fingers from top to bottom. Give the end of each toe a light squeeze.

Signal that the massage is coming to a conclusion by softly stroking the whole foot.

On to the hands. Furiously typing e-mails and text messages and fiddling with our PDAs (not to mention any old-fashioned writing or drawing you might do) gives our hands a serious workout. Try the following to give your hands a break—as an added bonus, these techniques can be done on yourself!

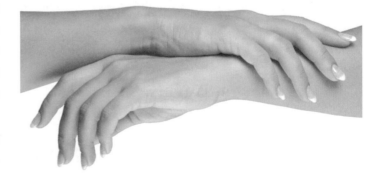

Begin by stretching the fingers by holding them together and gently pulling downward.

Massage the inside and outside of the hand using the thumb and the tips of the fingers. Massage each finger individually, moving from the base of the finger toward the end. Massage the space between each finger, including between the thumb and the index finger (this is actually a pressure point used in acupressure to relieve pain in the arm, shoulder, and neck). Knead the palm of the hand with the fist (as you did with the feet) and with the thumb. Finally, give something a good squeeze—from the edge of your desk to a soft "stress-relief" ball. Hold for about three seconds and release.

APPENDIX B: ESSENTIAL OILS AND THEIR HEALING PROPERTIES

Note: Not all of the oils in each category have properties listed because many of the properties of one oil apply to the others listed in that category.

Balancing oils:
- Bay Laurel
- Cedarwood
- Geranium—Especially good for oily and dull skin; antiseptic, fungicidal, cleansing, mildly pain-relieving, reduces inflammation; helps with stress and depression.
- Myrrh—Antiseptic, astringent, reduces inflammation, improves circulation, stimulates the regeneration of skin cells, assists in the healing of wounds; good for mature skin, chapped and cracked skin; cooling, calming, strengthening, increases mental clarity and focus.

Clarifying oils:

- Cypress
- Juniper
- Lemon—Also uplifting; can be used as an antidepressant or for stress relief.
- Peppermint—Anti-inflammatory, pain-relieving, antiseptic, astringent, relieves itching, stimulates circulation and can enliven dull, congested skin; clears the head, increases alertness, strengthens the nervous system.

Comforting oils:

- Bergamot—Antiseptic, anti-inflammatory, aids in the healing of wounds and scars; astringent. Uplifting and refreshing; it can help relieve anxiety and depression, ease grief and sadness, increase mental alertness; an effective insect repellant.
- Frankincense—Anti-inflammatory, antiseptic, astringent, helps wounds and scars to heal; good for dry and mature skin and wrinkles; sedative, warming, used for anxiety, nervous tension, and stress-related conditions.
- Melissa
- Rose—Along with jasmine, sandalwood, and ylang-ylang, it is considered an aphrodisiac.

Energizing oils:

- Eucalyptus—Analgesic, antiseptic, helps wounds to heal, used for burns, cuts, blisters. Centering, balancing, stimulating, used for exhaustion, congestive headaches.
- Grapefruit
- Lemongrass
- Rosemary—Antiseptic, gently pain-relieving, assists in the healing of wounds and scars; improves dull-looking skin and stimulates the scalp, promotes hair growth; clears the head, improves memory and concentration, reduces mental fatigue, combats headaches.

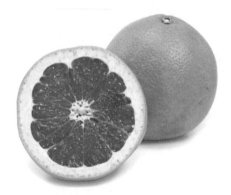

Focusing oils:

- Angelica
- Sweet basil—Clear and sweet aroma; sharpens concentration and has uplifting effects on depression.
- Jasmine samboc
- Lime

Sedating oils:

- Chamomile—Reduces inflammation; good for dry skin; calming, soothing, harmonizing; recommended for restlessness, anxiety; treats headaches and insomnia and improves memory.
- Clary Sage
- Marjoram—Pain-relieving, antiseptic, helps wounds to heal; comforting, soothing, strengthening; used for insomnia, headaches, stress.
- Patchouli

Uplifting oils:

- Lavender—Can be used as an antiseptic, to soothe minor cuts and burns, to calm and relax, and to soothe headaches.
- Orange/Mandarin
- Pine
- Tea Tree—Topical, anti-microbial properties; can be used as antiseptic and disinfectant.

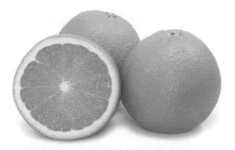

Appendix C: Glossary of Terms

Aromatherapy: the use of plant materials, called essential oils, and other scented compounds from plants for the purpose to affect one's mood or health. Aromatherapy is a general term that encompasses any of the many traditions that make use of essential oils, sometimes in conjunction with other alternative medical practices and spiritual beliefs.

Ayurveda: An ancient Indian system of preventive health care; the name means knowledge of life. According to this system, health is determined by harmony between three biological principles, called doshas: *vata*, which regulates movement; *pitta*, which regulates metabolism; and *kapha*, which regulates structure.

Chakra: A chakra (meaning wheel in Sanskrit) is a center of activity that receives, assimilates, and expresses life force energy. There are seven major chakras in the body, said to correspond with the basic states of consciousness, running in a straight line from the base of the spine to the top of the head. Chakras are believed to be a center of metaphysical and biophysical energy, and they must be as open as possible in order to function at their peak.

Chi (Qi): An important concept of traditional Chinese culture, chi is believed to be part of every living thing, as a kind of life force or spiritual energy (similar to the Ayurvedic principle of prana). It is often translated to mean energy flow, or literally as air or breath.

Essential oil: any of a class of volatile oils obtained from plants through distillation or extraction that has the scent and other characteristic properties of the plant; used mainly in the manufacture of perfumes, flavors, and pharmaceuticals.

Lymph: The lymphatic vessels branch into tissues throughout the body, similar to the circulatory system. Lymphatic vessels carry lymph, a colorless, watery fluid that comes from fluid in the tissues. The lymphatic system is an important part of the body's immune system. Lymph transports infection-fighting cells called lymphocytes throughout the body and is involved in the removal of foreign matter and cell debris.

Lymph drainage: A therapeutic massage technique that promotes and stimulates the lymphatic system, helping to move impurities out of the body.

Meridians: In traditional Chinese medicine, meridians are the invisible pathways in the body that circulate chi. There are 12 main meridians in the body, six yin and six yang, and each relates to one of the organs.

Prana: A Sanskrit word meaning breath. It refers to a vital, life-sustaining force of living beings and vital energy in natural processes of the universe that permeates everything.

Yin/Yang: In Chinese philosophy, yin and yang are the two opposing forces in the universe. Both are equal and necessary for harmony and health. Yang represents such principles as strong, active, bright, and male. Yin is weak, passive, dark, and female. The concept of the two forces is represented by a circle with interlinking black and white halves.

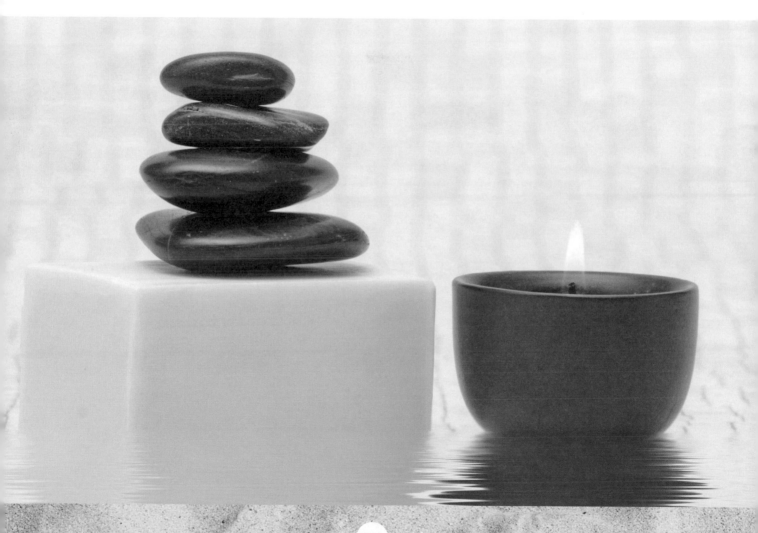

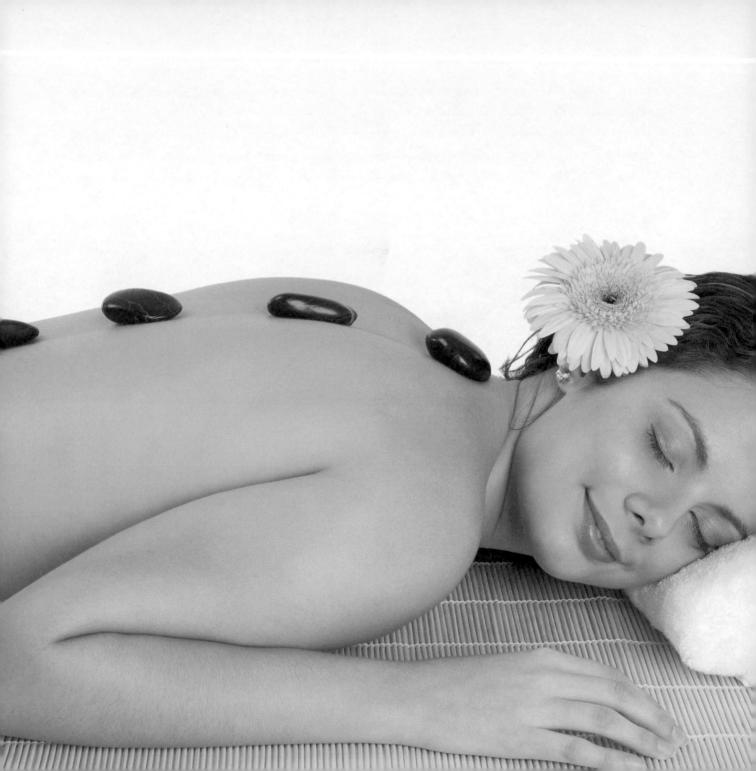

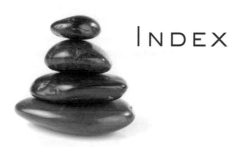

Index

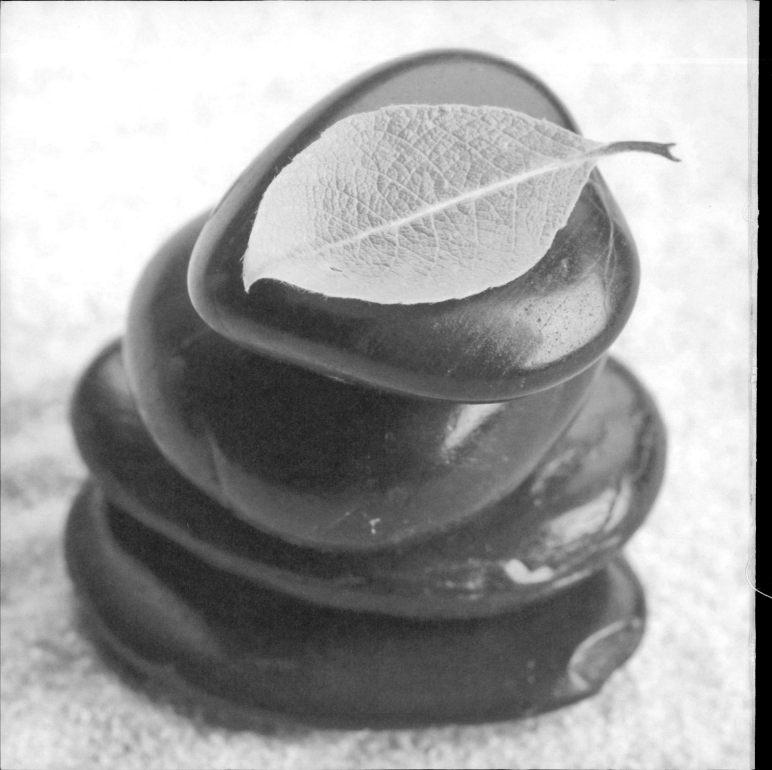